Residency Interview and Match

Real-Life Examples Tailored to Your Success

First Edition

Umesh Sharma, MD, PhD

Disclaimer

The ideas and information presented in this book are based on the author's current state of knowledge with best intention to help medical residency candidates. The author makes no express or implied representation that the strategies and information provided in this book are correct. The candidate names, faculty names, and geographical information mentioned in this book are arbitrary. Readers should check the most recent literature regarding current residency application guidelines, regulations, and interview procedure. The author does not accept any responsibility or liability for any errors in the text of this book.

To my wife, Sara, and my sons, Rosan and
Pratik

For your appreciation, encouragement, and endurance

Contents

Chapter 1

ECFMG, ERAS, and NRMP: What Do You Need to Know?

Chapter 2

A Brief Introduction to Residency Training in the USA

Chapter 3

Residency Training Structure: An Insider's Perspective

Chapter 4

Writing a Personal Statement

Chapter 11

Why Did I Write This Book?

After years of medical training, series of United States Medical Licensing Examination, time away from your family and friends, you have entered a critical juncture of your career transition. Sure, how you performed in your medical school, how your scores are, and how well rounded and confident you are in your communication and interpersonal skills will determine whether you can get into the residency of your choice. Nevertheless, with a dramatic increase in the volume of applicants and widening gap between the applicants and matched candidates year by year, it is becoming increasingly important that your application should be extremely well prepared.

A great residency application package includes a carefully written and goal-directed personal statement; strong and highly supportive letters of recommendation; and a clean, coherent, and consistent common application form. Once you are invited for the interview, it is equally important to understand what it means to be interviewed by the programs and what valuable information your potential residency programs are trying to extract from you. It is not all about how you dress, how you talk, and how you have scored in your USMLE. They are looking for a reliable trainee, a passionate teacher, and a dependable colleague. Your search for residency is not over even after you have completed your interviews. It is important that you appreciate what they have done for you thus far, and also, any further communication with the program directors (PDs) should not go shoddy.

Residency Interview and Match: Real-Life Examples Tailored to Your Success is a succinct but complete guide to help you chart through this process. The main purpose of this book is to provide you ample examples, complete with explanations, so that you actually understand what should be done and why it is done this way. Each of these examples are matched to your real-life stories so that you will quickly figure out which cohort you belong to and what it means to you to prepare for this application.

Finally, what you do as a medical student transitioning to become a physician makes me very proud. I have spoken to several of you in the classroom, in the wards, in the cafeteria, and occasionally in the pubs. The journey you have ventured earns great respect and does not deserve a tearful approach to prepare for your residency application. I hope this book will help you shape your application in a different and distinct way. Enjoy reading this book, and I wish you success in getting into the residency of your choice.

UCS

Chapter 1

ECFMG, ERAS, and NRMP: What Do You Need to Know?

Before you apply for your residency, it is very important to be aware of appropriate timelines, required documentation, time off from your education or work, and anticipated costs. For international medical graduates (IMGs, physicians who have obtained their medical degree outside the United States or Canada), the first step is to check whether you have fulfilled the minimal standards for eligibility for residency application. An Educational Commission for Foreign Medical Graduates (ECFMG) certification is a requirement for international medical graduates to enter residency training in the USA. For an ECFMG certification, candidates should pass the USMLE Step 1 and Step 2 CK (clinical knowledge) and CS (clinical skills) exams. Test of English as a Foreign Language is no longer a prerequisite for an ECFMG certification.

The Electronic Residency Application Service (ERAS) transmits your residency application, letters of recommendation, USMLE transcript, medical student performance evaluation, and other supporting documents to the individual programs you have applied to. ERAS has four components that work in coordination for your application to be successfully transmitted and downloaded by the individual programs.

MyERAS

This is the website you log in to using your Association of American Medical Colleges ID. Here you choose individual programs you are interested in and then assign your documents.

Dean's Office Workstation (DWS)

This is the software utilized by your medical school staff to create ERAS electronic token that you use to log in to MyERAS.

Program Director's Workstation (PDWS)

This is the software that individual programs use to download, sort, review, and rank your applications.

ERAS PostOffice

This is the central bank of the computers that transmit the information from your application and your dean's office to the individual programs you have applied to.

The National Resident Matching Program (NRMP) is an impartial venue for matching applicant's and programs' preferences for each other. Remember, NRMP does not process your application. It is critical that you register to NRMP, submit your rank order list (ROL), and, most importantly, *certify* it. NRMP will have no mercy on you if you forget to certify your ROL. You are expected to check the updated guidelines and details about residency application procedure on a regular basis. Of course, it is important to be familiar with an individual program's prerequisites before you transmit your application. Equally, individual states in the USA have different licensing requirements that programs are required to abide by.

It is common for the candidates to apply for more than one specialty. Of course, it depends on what exactly you would like to pursue as your career choice. In addition, there are certain advantages in applying for multiple specialties: the ERAS costs are calculated based on how many programs you have applied to. After the first ten programs, your cost starts increasing steeply. However, if you apply for two or more different specialties, you will be paying relatively less for the first ten programs regardless of how many you have applied to. Having said this, remember that it is very important to prepare your application package very carefully for each of those specialties you intend to apply for. Never send a generic personal statement. Never send a letter of recommendation to internal medicine if the LOR writer specifically states that you are interested in pediatrics. This only hurts your reasoning and credibility. Instead, you can ask your recommendation letter writers to comment on your knowledge, skills, abilities, attributes, and manners rather than describe what specialty you are interested in or suited for.

Chapter 2

A Brief Introduction to Residency Training in the USA

A resident typically works under the supervision of a fully licensed and mostly board-certified physician. Residency training is regulated by a body called the resident review committee (RRC). Residents are supposed to work and learn. In the old days, since majority of residents used to spend most of their time working in the hospital, i.e., working "in house," they were often referred to as house staff. Now the term "house staff" is used less commonly.

Most of the time, first-year residents are referred to as interns. Some programs refer to them as junior residents or lower-level residents. Second-year residents are referred to as residents or senior residents. Third-year residents are addressed as senior residents or graduating residents.

Internal medicine and pediatrics typically have three years of residency training. Pathology has two components—anatomical pathology and clinical pathology—and it takes a total of four years to complete both. It is highly unusual for a resident to pursue only one component of pathology training, but it does exist, at least in principle.

Some residents who have just completed their training decide to take an extra year of *chief residency* to develop teaching, leadership, and administrative skills. Chief residents make the work as well as the academic calendar for the rest of the residents. Chief residents work very closely with the program directors and the rest of the faculty members. Medical specialties that have a relatively smaller number of residents (e.g., pathology) do designate one or two of the senior residents as chief residents.

Some specialties need a transitional year before the start of the actual residency. For example, neurology needs a year of internal medicine training before actual neurology training can begin.

There is a separate training track that candidates with interest or background in research can pursue. This track is called the physician scientist track, or the clinical scientist track. Majority of university programs in the USA do enroll residents through this track. Most of the time, candidates who choose to pursue this track undergo a two-day interview procedure as opposed to one day only in categorical tracks. This extra day of interview allows candidates to speak to several faculty members from different divisions about their research interest. The faculty members will also rigorously test the candidates on what they are interested in and how they foresee themselves doing this research.

Different programs have their own style of evaluating and grading candidates' applications. Some programs develop a format with a scoring system, and candidates with satisfactory scores are invited for the interview. Many programs give relatively higher gravity to USMLE scores, whether the candidates passed at the first attempt and how recently the candidate has graduated out of medical school.

Please carefully check the criteria below before you apply to a program. No program director will invite you for interview if you do not clearly meet the requirements they have posted online.

The following components should be looked into when you are revising your application:

1. **Personal statement:** A personal statement stands as a critical determinant of the success of your application. This is the only component of your residency application that you can substantially change at this stage of the game plan. Personal

statement actually means a personal statement of your goals and objectives. Your goals can be short-term, long-term, or both. That means your statement should exclusively state what you are looking for in a program like the one you are applying to and how it fits with your own goals and objectives. Then you reason why you can be the most suitable candidate for this residency and how your previous experience and current work can be an asset in what you are expected to perform. You also explain what additional skills and attributes you have gained during your medical training that make you distinct from the rest of the applicants. A poorly written, incoherent, and goalless personal statement would be suicidal.

2. **Letters of recommendation:** Letters of recommendation are directly mailed out by the letter writers. So in a practical sense, you do not have control over the letters. Some busy mentors can sometimes ask you to write a draft letter. Realize that the draft you prepare may not be the

part of the letter that they mail out to ERAS. They can also ask you to e-mail your curriculum vitae to them. In any case, a strong letter is a major determinant of your success. You may e-mail your letter writers some sample letters for their reference if they are not very used to writing a letter of recommendation for residency. Clarify what is expected of such a letter and what areas of strength these letters should comment on to be of help in your application. However, an experienced letter writer will know the style and format of such letters and will likely not entertain the candidate making any specific demands or suggestions.

3. **USMLE scores:** Since this is a very objective evaluation of your medical knowledge, program directors would like to pay attention to your USMLE scores. These days, there are several of candidates score at 99th percentile. Then, it becomes necessary to review your three-digit score. Even if your scores are not exceptionally high, you still have a good chance of matching if you do well in other areas of evaluation. Making multiple

attempts is not admired, but many programs are open to consider such candidates for residency application.

4. **Dean's letter:** Most medical schools have a standard format for the dean's letter. Sometimes the dean's letter is written by an assistant or vice dean. This letter will comment on how you did during your medical training, where you stood among your batch mates, and what makes you unique among others. Any delay or difficulty in completing your medical training or any disciplinary actions taken against you is another area that this letter is supposed to comment on. If you have medical school awards or honors like membership in the Alpha Omega Alpha Honor Medical Society, this letter should clearly state this in its main content (preferably in boldface type).

5. **Number of years since your graduation:** This starts becoming relevant if you have graduated more than three years before you have started

applying for your residency. More than five years away from medical school is certainly an issue with many of the programs. Remember, most of the time, it is a state medical board, rather than a residency training program, that makes these decisions. Therefore, do not be adamant if a program has clearly listed these criteria as a prerequisite for your application.

6. **Clinical experience:** This is a bit fuzzy since clinical experience comes out of residency. For U.S. or Canadian graduates, this is normally not an issue. For international graduates, hands-on clinical experience is considered a plus. Many candidates manage to do some elective rotations in the USA while they are still enrolled in their medical school in their own country. This is great! But if you are not able to do so, you can, like many others, do externships (which allows them to learn how to take a patient's history and perform a physical exam) in different hospitals. Clinical observership is more of

an informal rotation and normally does not involve direct interaction with patients.

7. **Research, publications, presentations:** Research can be relevant only to some extent for community programs. However, if you have applied to bigger university-based programs with plenty of research backup, this component will have the highest gravity among all the components we have been discussing. Research means a careful clinical or bench research that has yielded some new data and has been presented in local or international meetings. If your abstract is submitted for review, you can still mention that your research is "under peer review." A review article is not counted as a research, but it is appreciated if you have made a substantial contribution to writing one. Meta-analyses of a good clinical relevance are perceived as research work. Your published articles should be presented in the correct format. For example,

Okita, K., T. Ichisaka, and S. Yamanaka. Generation of germline-competent

induced pluripotent stem cells. Nature
448 (2007): 313–317.

8. **Honors, awards, professional memberships:**
Several medical schools honor their students with
prizes, awards, and professional or honorary
memberships. These awards should be explicit in
your application. Remember, whenever you
mention a particular award, state also why this has
been awarded to you. For example, if you received
a professionalism award, then you have to explain
why this was given to you. For example,

   Professionalism award (2009):
   Designated to a final-year medical
   student who shows utmost empathy,
   respect, altruism, responsiveness, and
   determination to learn and teach.

9. **ECFMG status:** If you have not obtained an
ECFMG certificate yet because you have not
completed your USMLEs, you better start working
on that. Not having an ECFMG certificate makes

programs uncertain as to how you will do in the future and whether they can count on you as a potential candidate for their training program.

10. **Visa status**: If you are a U.S. citizen or a lawful permanent resident, it is time to look away now. Remember, there are certain visa types you can apply for. An H-1B visa allows you to do your residency in a worker status, and there is no home return requirement. A J-1 visa, although very attractive in terms of rapidity of its decision and ease of renewal, has a mandatory home return requirement. There are certain exceptions to this mandatory home return. It is important that you check the visa regulations and prerequisites before you apply for the residency of your choice. Further information can be obtained at www.uscis.gov.

Chapter 3

Residency Training Structure: An Insider's Perspective

Pathology Residency Training

There are several reasons why one would like to choose pathology as a career of choice. Pathology is a highly technical specialty with an enormous opportunity to develop and advance laboratory, surgical, and procedural competence. Pathologists are unique in the sense that they have a wealth of knowledge on the pathogenesis of disease; can formulate pertinent laboratory investigation plans; and are able to retrieve, process, and read pathology specimens.

Many of us think pathologists only look at slides and make a diagnosis for clinicians. Pathologists actually do way more than that. There are several branches of pathology, ranging from pure molecular and genetic pathology to medical examination and forensic pathology. Coroners are pathologists who are entrusted to perform postmortem examination of a body. Surgical pathologists read frozen sections and analyze gross and microscopic slides of tissue samples for diagnosis. Cytopathologists are adept with fine needle aspiration cytology and mostly deal with the cellular aspect of pathology. Blood banking deals with blood transfusion and transfusion reactions. Molecular and genetic pathologists examine, analyze, and troubleshoot complex genetic analyses (e.g., HLA typing) and biomolecular techniques.

Pathology is becoming an increasingly popular field these days for the following main reasons: 1) it allows a flexible lifestyle, 2) it offers reasonable compensation, 3) it is a profession guided by in-depth understanding of the disease process, 4) it offers better research opportunities, and 5) it provides higher chances of receiving competitive research grants.

From a residency application standpoint, your personal statement should be clear and explicit on what you expect to learn out of a great pathology training program. (Remember, most of the pathology training programs are university based, and they normally have three to six spots on average.) You would also like to reason why you would be the best fit for a pathology residency. This reasoning should be backed up by your previous track record showing your interest in laboratory medicine and pathology.

More recently, it has become obvious that physicians with background in basic science are more attracted to pathology. However, it is not mandatory to have a laboratory or research experience before you can apply for a pathology residency. Certainly, you would not like to write a nonspecific personal statement and send totally pathology-unrelated letters of recommendation to apply for pathology residency. The professional spirit of pathologists is high and deep, and they will be willing to work with colleagues with the same level of desire and determination to learn and improve.

Anesthesia Residency Training

A lot of times, medical students wonder what exactly it is that anesthetists do. This happens because many medical schools in the USA and elsewhere do not mandate anesthesia rotation for the completion of medical school training. A typical candidate who applies for anesthesia training would need to have persistence, passion, and perseverance to learn and deliver what is expected of him or her. Unlike physicians with other specialties, anesthetists are required to be compulsive in interrogation and retrieving in-depth clinical information, and bold and unambiguous in clinical decision making.

As an anesthetist, you will be challenged with a diversity of cases ranging from a minor elective surgery in an otherwise-healthy person to a fragile elderly gentleman with a myriad of clinical problems whose chances of pulling through a procedure are slim. You may also encounter a baby, a child, a pregnant female, a trauma patient, a cancer patient, et cetera, et cetera. You will encounter anyone! Since you will not have direct admitting responsibility, you will always be treated as a consultant.

From the resident training perspective, anesthesia training will take four years. Out of those four years, the first year is a transitional year. The transitional year is often coordinated with the internal medicine residency program of your own institution. Some candidates prefer to do a transitional year in a separate place while transferring to anesthesia as a PGY-2.

Of note, anesthesia training offers a more flexible lifestyle and has ample opportunities for specialization in advanced fields of medicine like regional anesthesia, pain management, critical care, etc. It is sometimes heard that anesthetists are treated as a subsidiary member of the surgical team and not given enough respect or due regard by the surgeons. Many other anesthetists disagree with this. It is not up to us to change someone else's manners or professional skills, but there should be no doubt in anyone's mind that anesthetists absolutely do not play an inferior role to anyone else in any of the clinical encounters they are consulted upon.

Dermatology Residency Training

Dermatology counts as a competitive residency to get into because of the limited number of slots they offer, the ease and cleanliness of the training, and the relatively less hectic schedule, along with admirable compensation. Good news for the dermatology candidates: not too many candidates, especially international medical graduates, apply for dermatology residency. Dermatology residency will require a year of internship, which you can complete in the same institution or somewhere else. If you are interested in pediatric dermatology, internship in pediatrics will make better sense.

It is important to identify your interest during your fourth year in medical school. Speak to the dermatology faculty members and program directors and tell them why dermatology intrigues you the most. You will probably not want to raise the issues of work hours, compensation, or call schedule. The reason for not doing this is that the program directors may feel that you should have developed a better vision about your residency and have set up your priorities differently.

It can sometimes be difficult to secure a dermatology spot, especially if you do not have Alpha Omega Alpha membership, outstanding USMLE scores, and exceptional LORs written by established senior faculties. Probably it is a better idea to have a backup plan handy. Some programs also offer research fellowship in dermatology. You might want to consider doing a year of research before reapplying for dermatology residency.

Dermatologists should have sharp eyes, a quick brain, a fresh look, and a positive attitude. Your attending will rigorously test your readiness, aptitude, and attitude toward dermatology during the interview. There is no right or wrong answer; but remember, whoever is able to clearly articulate his or her goals and objectives and,has a plan for the future and a track from the past will possibly secure a spot in dermatology.

Emergency Medicine Residency Training

Emergency medicine residency has just completed its teenage. Within this relatively short period, EM has earned substantial repute and character and has raised interest among many medical graduates. Most of the EM residency programs last three years. Three-year programs have fewer electives but more hard-core emergency medicine, and are appropriate if you are willing to run your career more as a clinician rather than a researcher. Four-year programs are slightly laid-back and have plenty of electives and research time. You may typically choose an academic career after completing the four-year track.

Emergency medicine residency training has many unique characteristics that others lack. It has a shift-based work schedule published mostly a month in advance. Your work hours are flexible, interchangeable with your colleagues', and sometimes can be really light (depending on which hospital you are working at). However, emergency medicine is a highly dynamic area of medicine that requires quick thinking, immediate action, multitasking, leadership skills, and resilience. On several occasions, you may need to face the unexpected, and a situation can change or turn berserk in no time, mainly in inner-city hospital ERs.

Emergency medicine also offers plenty of research opportunities, especially because there is ample opportunity for data gathering. EM has access to all the clinical and laboratory data obtained at the point of care. This makes the emergency department a rich place to retrieve and analyze original clinical database and formulate effectiveness of the existing investigation plan or treatment strategy.

If you are planning to apply for emergency medicine residency, plan in advance, identify your mentor, and obtain one to two letters of recommendations. The LORs should exclusively state how you have prepared yourself to get into emergency medicine residency and, based on your track record, how much you promise for the future. Your answers during the interview should be direct, straight, goal oriented, and honest. Get ready to answer what you would like to do after you are done with your residency. Know whether you are a community hospital kind of person or would rather work in an academic setting. Have your goals; discern your dreams. Finally, have persistence and perseverance in e-mailing the program, schedule your interview early, and write meaningful thank-you letters, rather than a sentence stating, "I thoroughly enjoyed that day." Having done all this, have fun on your match day.

Obstetrics and Gynecology Residency Training

Obstetrics and gynecology residency offers a rare and unique blend of outpatient vs. inpatient, medical vs. surgical, and routine vs. emergent care of female patients. The residency training typically lasts for four years; and again, like any other residency trainings, you can choose to work in a community hospital or in an academic or university hospital. Over the last many years, the scale of competition for OB-GYN residency has not changed substantially, but realize that OB-GYN is a fairly well-sought-after residency training. The main reason why medical graduates prefer OB-GYN is its unique variety and possibility to further specialize in quite advanced and fascinating areas of maternal and fetal medicine. Reproductive health, maternal and fetal medicine, pelvic reconstructive surgery, gynecologic oncology, etc., are a few areas of OB-GYN that attract physicians of high caliber and stance.

There is no secret formula for securing a spot for OB-GYN. Your desire and determination should manifest right from your third year. Have a firm mind-set, identify your interest, stay interested, and be visible. During your clerkship, do not hesitate to ask questions and contribute as much as you can. Enjoy your rotation, have coffee with the residents, ask them how their weekend went, etc. Do not come up with too many personal requisites during this training because OB-GYN is a branch of medicine that requires enormous time commitment, tenacity, and an ability to dedicate substantial amount of personal and family time for patient care.

Your personal statement should be essentially personal. Generic statements are detrimental, if not suicidal, to your application. Be clear why you want to do OB-GYN residency, what you expect out of any residency, and what makes you the best fit for the program you are applying to. Include your life experience (good or bad), and share an event, if any, that completely changed your mind-set. For example, if you have worked with an astute OB-GYN physician who treated his or her patients in such a way that you started envisioning yourself as a physician of similar caliber, mention this in your personal statement. Remember, personal statements are written by you, a real person and a human being, not by a strange supercreature.

Once you start getting invitations for an interview, respond promptly. Schedule early interviews and have ample interviews done so that your rank order list does not look too truncated. Always write follow-up e-mails, even if you don't get any response from the faculties. Do not forget to certify your rank order list. After you have done this, have fun on your match day and enjoy your residency.

Pediatrics Residency Training

What can I say that adequately describes the spirit and charisma of pediatrics? If you are planning on doing a pediatrics residency, you stand prominent among the rest of the candidates because of your desire to dedicate your profession to taking care of babies and children. You have already decided on making a long-term relationship with your patients and their families, and you have chosen a path toward a great deal of happiness and professional satisfaction watching how your patients feel better and how they grow.

If you believe that the biggest joy in life is having a healthy child, and are focused and motivated to work hard (as a team member and as a team leader), and do not hesitate to make bold decisions even if that might bring tears to someone's eyes, pediatrics is for you.

Pediatrics is not a mini-internal medicine, because babies and children are not simply micro-adults. It is an independent and well-rounded clinical specialty that offers you almost-endless opportunities to work with neonates, babies, children, and adolescents. "Caring for the caregiver" is a unique motto embraced by pediatricians who spend a substantial part of their clinical encounter speaking to their patients' family members.

If you are interested in a pediatrics residency, define your goal by your third year in medical school. Develop a habit of communicating with children and their parents. Carry a stethoscope with a little toy wrapped around it, so that the little one can happily play with it while you examine him or her. Some students also wear children-friendly apparels, but do not overdo it.

Your personal statement should be very fluent and congruous with your goals and objectives. Mention why you like pediatrics so much, explain how you have prepared yourself to be a pediatrician, and state what makes you different from other adult-oriented doctors. Your letter writers should be given ample amount of time to prepare and mail out your LOR.

Pediatrics offers a viable option for multiple fellowships— e.g., cardiology, gastroenterology, hematology-oncology, critical care, rheumatology, etc. If you are completely decided to get into a particular fellowship, then sharpen your goals in a way that they lead you toward achieving the fellowship of your choice. If you are not decided, then be honest and state that you have not yet come to a conclusion.

Schedule all your interviews early enough; write strong thank-you letters to make your presence felt. Admire what pediatricians do and be grateful for the invitation they have extended to you for an interview. Be responsive and appear responsible in your conversations. Finally, do not forget to call your friends to share your happiness with them on the match day!

Psychiatry Residency Training

If you have chosen to pursue psychiatry as a career, then you probably have a passion for extended communication and elaborate data entry and documentation, and an interest in the psychosocial aspect of your patient's life. You probably intend to have a strong and long-term relationship with your patients. In addition, pharmacotherapy and counseling are a few other areas of psychiatry that attract many candidates to this area.

Like any other residency, psychiatry has options for further specialization in more advanced areas like pediatric psychiatry, consultation and liaison, etc. Psychiatry is preferred by some candidates because of its more flexible lifestyle, reasonable compensation, and the possibility of having one's own practice without much difficulty. Patients tend to be more faithful to their psychiatrists in general, most likely because psychiatrists put in time and effort to address their patients' physical, mental, and social well-being.

Applying for a psychiatry residency should not be painful as long as you have put worthy efforts into writing your personal statement and identifying enthusiastic letter writers. Do not write a generic personal statement if you are applying for psychiatry because there is nothing generic about it. Furthermore, the program director will have enough insight to read and decipher your interest while he or she reads your personal statement. Enthusiasm is hard to create if you are not enthusiastic about doing psychiatry.

Like many other residencies, you are expected to do four years of training. You will need a great deal of patience to take an accurate and extended clinical history. Your first year can roughen up a bit because you will be spending three to four months with internal medicine residents. You can as well balance your training by splitting these months between internal medicine and emergency medicine. But many psychiatry residents enjoy this moment, and some rare ones actually seek to continue with internal medicine. Your second year will be focused on inpatient psychiatry, and when you reach the more senior years, you will spend more time doing outpatient psychiatry and providing consulting services. Certainly there is no hard-and-fast rule on how you should be trained, as your program director can make necessary adjustments based on your training requirements.

During the interview, you will certainly be asked why you would like a career in psychiatry. Have a really well-phrased answer handy. Know your short-term as well as long-term goals and be clear on whether you would like to work in a community hospital or in an academic center, and why. If you have given your best shot and have not forgotten to certify your rank order list, you can expect to match to the program of your choice. There will be exceptions, but exceptions are neither major nor minor criteria for your decision making.

Family Medicine Residency Training

Whether you visit a busy inner-city hospital or a sophisticated suburban clinic, you will get a taste of a family physician. Realize that more than 90 percent of common illnesses do not need to be evaluated or treated by specialists. Although there is an increasing tendency to redundantly refer patients to advanced specialty for rather small reasons, family physicians are the ones who can make a real difference, quickly and appropriately in a majority of cases.

The other aspect of family medicine training is that it is very well rounded and encompasses multiple disciplines of medicine like internal medicine, general surgery, pediatrics, obstetrics and gynecology, psychiatry, mental health, etc. Since the residency typically lasts for three years, it is impossible to acquire extensive theoretical and practical acumen in each of these specialties. But, family physicians understand enough to do enough to save lives.

In a typical outpatient setting, where there is heterogeneity of patient population, no one performs better than family physicians, because of the assortment of clinical training they have received and the experience they have gained. Great news: family medicine residency is not far from possible to secure if you have made a sincere effort to get one. Your personal statement should explicitly explain why you chose family medicine over others. Remember, if you are willing to focus in specialties like cardiology, gastroenterology, oncology, etc., family medicine is not for you. But if you have a decent interest in pursuing a career in sport medicine, women's health, faculty transition and training, etc., then you will be eligible for a fellowship tailored to your interest and your need.

There are certain hospitals in the USA that are run largely by family physicians. Those hospitals will offer you a very wide and inclusive clinical exposure during your training. Always set your goals; know how you see yourself after five years and ten years (an experienced physician, teacher, researcher, sports physician, faculty member, etc.). Remember, your priorities and goals can change, pretty much the way many things change in life; but this does not mean you should not have any right from the start. After the interview, promptly write thank-you letters and reply to any e-mails you have received from the program. You can also voluntarily ask them whether you can be of any assistance and provide your cell phone number to the program co-coordinator. Having said this, there are chances that some of the family medicine residency training slots can sometimes go unmatched. Therefore, if you think it is necessary, get ready for the scramble.

Ophthalmology Residency Training

Ophthalmology is not only a very competitive residency training to get into, but it also has a slightly different temporal setup for application, interviews, and matching. It is an early-match specialty for which you have to complete the application by the end of August (when you are doing your fourth year). They will then invite you for an interview, which typically takes place in October, November, and December.

Typically, candidates tend to apply to forty to fifty programs. Since ophthalmology is a competitive residency to get into, it is important to have your credentials carefully assembled before you apply. Your letter writers should believe that you have enough desire and motivation to pursue ophthalmology as your career choice, and this should be explicit in their letters. Try to have a letter from the chief of ophthalmology division at your school (he or she is a chief for a reason!). The dean's letters will be released on November 1, and certainly, program directors will be looking into what you have accomplished, where you stand, and how you have performed during your medical training. No need to mention that your USMLE scores are important, but I have spoken to some PDs who do not really care about the scores but instead weigh an individual's overall scholastic ability, including research and publications. Anyway, having better scores does not hurt.

After you receive an invitation for an interview, do not wait too long to schedule it. Many programs interview candidates only on certain days, and it is not unusual that those slots get filled quickly. Dress professionally, speak softly, and be considerate and nonjudgmental. You are competing with a small subset of candidates who have faith and passion for getting into this most competitive residency training. Promptly send nongeneric thank-you letters and respond to programs' queries quickly and adequately. Schedule a second look if you think that helps you.

Ophthalmology residency training programs require a year of internship or a transitional year in accredited residency programs. This year can be completed in internal medicine, pediatrics, or, rarely, surgery. It might help to do your transitional training within the premises of the place where you are going to do your ophthalmology residency, but it is your choice.

Internal Medicine Residency Training

So here is the most popular and diverse part of training—internal medicine. Internal medicine, on its own, is a well-demanded and to some extent well-reimbursed specialty. You have multiple routes to choose from on what you would like to do as your career choice. You can stay as a primary care physician or move on to start fellowship training in a specialty of your choice.

Upon completion of internal medicine training, you are eligible to start your fellowship in one of the following areas: cardiology, gastroenterology, pulmonary/critical care, hematology-oncology, nephrology, physical therapy and rehabilitation, allergy and immunology, endocrine, rheumatology, infectious diseases, etc. No doubt, internal medicine residency training is well mixed and well rounded. Many candidates worry that internal medicine is a very demanding specialty in terms of time commitment. They also fear that night calls are as frequent as Q3 and can be brutal. That is correct to some extent, but internal medicine has several elective rotations that have no night-call responsibilities. Also, it is common to have one or two research rotations during your training. Research rotations can be utilized either to do a focused and goal-oriented research or simply to review literature and write a review article and perform a meta-analysis of existing literature.

Internal medicine training lasts for three years. If you have chosen a research (or physician scientist) track, this can be extended to four years. It all depends on what you would like to pursue as your career choice. If you are OK practicing in a primary care setting in a community hospital, probably you will not need an additional year of research training. But if you intend to become a faculty member in a big academic center and want to establish a meaningful track of clinical or biomedical research, then you will benefit from an academic training track.

For those who want to apply for fellowship training, you should apply during the second year of your residency. Typically, application cycles start in December. There are some fellowships that are more competitive than others.

Internal medicine is a competitive residency, but since there are large numbers of training slots, there is a good chance that you will be able to secure one. Apply early and schedule your interviews right away. Remember, they interview hundreds of candidates for ten to twenty training slots more than an average program offers. They are crammed with lots of things; and the last thing they will appreciate is you becoming their distracter because of your inflexible schedule, incomplete documents, or too many phone calls or e-mails for minor issues. Be prompt and direct and show your flexibility. Be respectful to the program coordinators; make sure they can reach you without difficulty.

During the interview, stay motivated and answer questions in a simple and predictable way. Do not flip-flop your goals based on who you are speaking to. If you are not sure, state that you are having a learning curve. Do not forget to send thank-you letters; you can send one to the program coordinator as well. Answer PD's e-mails promptly if he or she gets back to you. Remember, you do not need to reply to all the generic e-mails, though. If you have made this effort, of course supported by strong LORs and personal statement, you are thriving well to match to a program of your choice.

Surgery Residency Training

Have you decided to pursue a career in surgery? Do you firmly believe that the field of surgery can fit your way of your life? If you answered yes to these two questions with a determinate mind, surgery residency is for you. Rest assured that you are about to enter an extremely challenging but rewarding area of medical practice. Practicing surgery as a surgeon is different from training yourself as a resident of surgery. There will be instances when you will need to rush to the operating theater in the middle of the night. There will be more instances that you will feel tired and fatigued and a bit frustrated.

Then why do people choose this? Well, if you are a surgeon, you are a species of passion and perseverance, and you do not shy away from challenges. You are firm, determinate, commanding, and probably swifter than anyone in making quick and life-saving decisions. You don't fear nights, and you do not run away from challenges. Patients and their families appreciate what you do!

It is important to realize that preparing for a surgery residency application is a harbinger of your real residency.

This process can be very intense at times. Right from your third year in medical school, start thinking about what will be the best fit for you—otolaryngology, plastic surgery, vascular surgery, etc. It also helps if you do rotations at surgical ICUs to have a firsthand glimpse of severe and sometimes life-threatening surgical conditions like burn, trauma, ruptured aneurysm, etc.

Spend ample time to prepare your CV and write a personal statement. Your goals and perspectives should be clear in your statement. Never, ever, send a generic personal statement if you are seriously willing to become a surgeon. Even if you are applying for a preliminary position, exert your best efforts to prepare a compelling application package. Your letter writers should be aware of the fact that you are applying for competitive residency training that demands enormous mental and physical stamina to successfully complete it. They should comment on your abilities and skills on that ground. Sure, you need to provide them ample time, but do not forget to send them a reminder if needed.

Once you have submitted your application, be alert as to how things are being perceived by the program. Check whether they have downloaded your documents. If there is something you have sent that is not downloaded, something has gone wrong. Call ERAS and figure out what happened. What if your letter writers never sent a letter for you? There is no hard-and-fast rule on how many programs you can apply to, but it is your decision. If you have a stellar application package and you are flawless in your interview skills, you may easily get what you wish for. On average, some forty applications is not a bad idea.

On the day of the interview, dress formally and reasonably. Be humble but firm while you communicate. Do not flip-flop in your goals. Do not raise the issue of reimbursement or malpractice. Have a constructive communication; discuss your family circumstances and clarify if you have special needs. You do not want to have regrets in the middle of your residency just because you decided not to share the fact that your wife also needed an internship training in the same area, the same year.

After your interviews are done, promptly send thank-you letters, and you should be available to answer any queries the program coordinator or PD might have in the course of their decision making. Finally, do not forget to certify your rank order list. Good luck.

Chapter 4

Writing a Personal Statement

The personal statement is probably the most important factor to impact the outcome of your application at this stage. Remember, it is *your* personal statement, and it speaks about *you*. An English-language editor or a gifted writer may not understand the hardships you have gone through and may not have faced the challenges you have faced. So who writes the best personal statement for you? The correct answer is *you*.

Before you start writing your personal statement, think about this: Well, what makes me different from others? Why am I writing this personal statement? What intrigued me about becoming a doctor? How have I nurtured my interest since then? What unique life experiences do I have that makes me distinct from others? What hardships and struggles have I faced, and how was I able to overcome them? How did I develop my resilience and stamina?

A boring, incorrect, and generic personal statement is often detrimental to your application.

Your personal statement is also a platform for you to highlight your personal attributes, moral values, and family beliefs. This makes your personal statement truly personal.

Equally, you may explain why you have certain shortcomings in your applications. For example, if you defended your PhD dissertation (successfully) around the time you took your clinical skills exam (unsuccessfully!), then your second attempt may not be an issue for ranking your application.

The following are some mistakes to avoid while writing your personal statement: solely describing your curriculum vitae, making multiple grammatical errors, conflicting statements, self-exaggeration, presenting yourself as a granddad figure, and arrogance hidden inside high USMLE scores. After you are done writing your statement, it is preferable to ask a nonmedical person to take a look at it. Do not cram it with the facts and advices obtained from too many people, as too many cooks will spoil the broth.

Family Medicine

I chose family medicine over other specialities of medicine not because I was looking for a challenge-free, laid-back, but financially rewarding career. This decision came out of my own belief and passion—a passion shaped by my personal and family life and the belief imparted by the community where I lived and grew up.

I compare my work to what I do in my day-to-day life. When I see a two-year-old child strolled over by his seventy-two-year-old grandmother and accompanied by his pregnant mother and eleven-year-old sister, I identify the concept of a family. This brings out the true love driven by selfless motivation to help and nurture. As a family physician, I envisage myself as one of this family, one of such many families.

What can I compare to a branch of medicine that allows me to serve and learn from practically any one and every one of the society? What would give me better satisfaction than to develop an everlasting relation of trust and care? What would give me more pleasure than to educate a child about the importance of oral hygiene? What would be more rewarding than to remind a fifty-year-old gentleman to undergo colon cancer screening? Sometimes, I think, each of us should become a family physician!

Have I prepared myself to be a suitable candidate for family medicine residency? Well, what would make a suitable candidate? I know that when surgeons remove gallstones, they garner a great deal of thankfulness. A urologist scraps the enlarged prostate, allowing urine to flow, and gets praised as an angel. Sure, it helps someone! But who has been a lifelong friend of this seventy-two-year-old gentleman whose prostate has grown out of control recently? Who returns his phone calls in the middle of the night when he was not able to pass urine? Who would again continue to see this gentleman after he is discharged out of the urologist's practice? I would like to! I would be honoured to! This is what makes me think that I am more than prepared to start this residency training.

My personality and my previous track of working with developmentally challenged children make me a determinate individual whose only interest is to get involved in care. Care means mutual understanding, kindness, a desire to solve problems, and, more importantly, an ownership of one's responsibility. Sometimes they see care being compared to a rigid language, formality and rituals. Well, not me as family physician! No us as the residents of family medicine! Not the hospital I will be doing my residency at. Not my program director! Because we are different—we care to make a

we care to make a difference by impacting
our patient's life, both at personal & family level

difference; we positively impact our patient's life, and both at

personal and family levels.

Many thanks in anticipation for your considerations, and I look

forward to hearing from you soon.

Internal Medicine

"If you seek a life free of books, pagers and germs, you should probably think of something else." I remember the reaction of my best friend after he recognized my ambition to become a physician. Although I stumbled initially during this decision-making process, I nurtured this dream ever since I saw people constantly waiting outside the small suburban hospital of my hometown. How a doctor who is no different from all of us can understand our pain and suffering and can relieve us of them was the mystery that occupied my mind. I grew up in a community with a very high doctor-to-population ratio, and seeing a physician was like witnessing the blue moon; becoming one was close to impossible. However, after I graduated from my high school with honors, I was selected into one of the pioneer medical schools of my country after a vigorous competition.

After completing the first two years of my medical education, I started my internal medicine rotations. I still remember my first case as a medical student—a young man with a rheumatic heart disease who suffered shortness of breath while returning home from his school. His friends brought him to ED while he was still in his school uniform. I listened to his heart and noticed the turbulence of blood flow. I just continued thinking, Why him? Why anyone? I looked at his eyes and could see his inner desire and determination to get better and get back to school, so that he could complete his study and relieve the financial hardship his parents had been facing. That day, I left the hospital answerless, confused, and alarmed. However, as time passed, I began to enjoy the challenge of correlating my theoretical acumen with patient interaction to come up with a successful diagnosis.

My experience of doing research and traveling to several different nations in Europe has in many ways helped me understand several unique aspects of human culture, beliefs, and struggles. I have learned to find the points of common interest and have developed a strong sense of *us* rather than *them.* My goals during this residency training are to develop strong clinical knowledge, understand the U.S. health care system, and develop into a critical thinker and investigator. I would also like to impart to those around me the tradition of great teaching initiated by my professors who selflessly helped me become a good doctor and a better human being.

In your residency program, I am looking forward to developing clinical knowledge and skills while working as a team member in a friendly environment with people from different social and cultural backgrounds. My desire to pursue the finest residency program in the world brings me to this land of opportunities. The dedication, determination, and perseverance that I put into my training will certainly help me achieve my goals and objectives. Now, I am more than ever determined to follow this path to be a compassionate and competent physician. I sincerely hope that you will consider my application positively.

Pathology

I believe a successful treatment begins with a correct diagnosis. During medical school, many cases influenced my decision to pursue pathology training. Many cases touched me; one in particular occurred early in my fourth year. I had had the opportunity to take care of a twelve-year-old boy named Teddy. In his twelve years, Teddy experienced many hardships. He came from a broken home, was one of six children, and had just lost his mother to AIDS. Teddy was suffering from worsening anemia that could not be cured with multiple transfusions. Most striking was the lack of answer as to its cause, despite multiple invasive procedures, including bone marrow biopsy. Many pediatricians, internists, and others attempted to solve this diagnostic puzzle without success. Finally, a brilliant pathologist ordered a peripheral blood sample. Upon seeing the blood smear, he remembered a similar case from years earlier. He knew to ask if the patient had recently visited the neighboring country of Nigeria, and he had. The pathologist, with his trained eye and armed with the data from previous workups and clinical experience, accurately diagnosed plasmodium falciparum–induced malaria, and Teddy was cured of his life-threatening illness. Ever since then, my interest in pathology has only been growing. During my residency, I have witnessed several similar cases where the patients have been crucially helped by astute pathologists. My experience as a pathology resident has always been gratifying.

I believe that my prior education and work experience have provided me with an excellent background to withstand the challenges of completing a pathology residency. My past research was focused on the pathogenesis of high blood pressure–induced end-organ damage, particularly in the heart and kidney. My research experience in molecular biology not only boosted my theoretical knowledge but also increased my practical skills, such as immunohistochemical studies, real-time polymerase chain reaction, and laser capture microdissection, which have facilitated and enhanced my learning process. My previous interactions with many clinicians and pathologists have helped me see the field of pathology from a broader perspective and strengthened my interest in this field. They have made me realize that a career in pathology can fulfill my ultimate goal of actively participating in patient care while keeping abreast of developments in academic medicine.

To develop a satisfactory profession, which allows continuous learning and making contributions to patient care and medical research, I am applying to continue my residency training in your program. In addition to a family-oriented reason, several other factors, including my academic track record, emphasis on research, and, most importantly, the rigorous training offered by your program remain the subject of my prime motivation. I strongly hope you will consider my request positively.

Pediatrics

My past experience has uniquely prepared me for a residency in pediatrics. I was born in a remote village in Montana. Although my mother never had the opportunity to go to school, she had great hopes for me and always encouraged me to get educated. Despite the fact that the girls in my community were not destined to go to school, I have come this far because of my three strengths: determination, perseverance, and self-confidence. My greatest desire was to go to college, study medical science, and eventually become a doctor. In this venture of life, I have learned to deal with numerous adversities, and, I believe, this experience has strengthened my ability to become a good physician.

My reasons for pursuing a career in pediatrics are numerous. The field offers a unique combination of primary care and teaching. Primary care allows for continuity of care leading to the development of trust, long-term relationships, and the delivery of comprehensive quality care. Also, as a pediatrician, I will have the opportunity to care for children of all ages and be involved in their physical and mental development starting from the day they are born. As a mother of a two-year-old, I have learned how challenging and rewarding it could be to become a successful pediatrician. Moreover, each child is a unique human being, and

[Each person is unique &]

each of them will provide me a learning opportunity at all phases of my career.

My career goals include enrolling in a residency program that will expose me to a diverse patient population and provide me with ample opportunities to obtain the training and skills that a competent pediatrician needs. I look forward to getting involved in research opportunities so that I can contribute to the exciting and rapidly growing field of pediatrics research. Although the broad field of pediatrics intrigues me the most, I will consider completing a fellowship in neonatology after I have had some experience as a house staff. I intend to make teaching part of my career, as a way for me to continue my academic, clinical, and personal growth.

Teaching

Chapter 5

Request for Letters of

Recommendation

It is important to identify your LOR writers at least four months before you submit your application. So what constitutes identifying your LOR writers? First, your LOR writers should have adequate knowledge about your clinical skills, and they should, at least partly, be aware of your professional and ethical behavior. Second, your LOR writers should be eager and willing to support your residency application. Third, you should feel confident that your LOR writer will manage to send a great supporting letter for you within the time frame you have stated. Fourth, your LOR writer should at least be a junior faculty member or an emeritus. Do not ask your fellow trainees to write an LOR for you.

Once you have identified your LOR writers, either personally speak to them or send them an e-mail. Now it is your last opportunity to persuade your LOR writers to write great things about you. Explain to them what you intend to do, what your goals are, and how you came to this conclusion. State that their help at this critical point of your career transition will be highly appreciated.

On many occasions, your LOR writers may not have enough knowledge on the style or format of such letters. Please refer to the next chapter for some sample LORs that your LOR writers may find helpful. If your LOR writers remain silent for weeks, do not hesitate to send them a reminder e-mail. It is safe to identify four to five letter writers so that if one of them cannot make it on time, you still have enough LORs to proceed with your application.

Sample 1

Dear Dr. Wellington,

I hope you are well and everything is going great at Western University, Department of Medicine. We are very excited by the fact that you will be giving us a lecture regarding the role of biomarkers for early detection of anemia.

Dr. Wellington, after a lot of thinking and deliberation, I have come to the conclusion that I will apply for internal medicine residency. Given my interest in the area of SLE and the research work I did investigating the organ specificity of different autoantibodies, I believe I will be able to help patients and continue doing research in this field. More than that, internal medicine has touched my personal life in a much more intimate way, as my granddad died of autoimmune hemolytic anemia and my grandma suffered from rheumatoid arthritis for more than twenty-five years.

During my internal medicine clerkship with you, I have found myself to be very confident in patient management, I have made several friends from different parts of the world, and have earned a lot of regard and respect for what I have done in the past. I am grateful to you for creating this learner-friendly and academically productive environment. I personally feel that my residency application will not be complete without your help. While I will always need your moral support and encouragement, I would also like to request for a letter of recommendation from you regarding my application. I do understand your busy schedule, but this will significantly enhance my career pathway.

I thank you in anticipation for your help, and I am looking forward to your reply. I am attaching my CV to this e-mail. Kindly let me know if I can be of any further assistance. I check my e-mails regularly and will get back to you promptly.

Sample 2

Dear Dr. Richardson,

Hope your clinical as well as research work is going fine. I have to apologize for such a long spell before writing to you. This year, I am applying for internal medicine residency training in the USA. My wife has already started doing family medicine residency in Atlanta, and my two-year-old son, Ricky, goes to an early learning center located in an Atlanta suburb. We also bought a small condominium and so far have remained kind of happy. I often communicate with Dave regarding our GI bleeding study and have heard from him that things are well in your department.

Dr. Richardson, I am submitting my residency application via ERAS very soon. I would like to humbly request you for a letter of recommendation. I have been performing well in internal medicine, and the dean has written a great letter for me. A letter from you will make my application extremely strong. I know you are busy fulfilling your responsibilities. Therefore, I have attached a template for you (just for the style).

Greetings to Romero, Guarrez, and others working there.

Thank you for your help.

Sample 3

Dear Dr. Smith,

Hope this e-mail finds you great. I am writing you from Portland, Oregon, where I am doing a brief clinical clerkship in the department of internal medicine at a local hospital.

After completing medical school, I was in a kind of dilemma whether to go for pathology or to have a more clinically interactive training in family medicine. The biggest drive for me to do family medicine was that if I decide to get back to Puerto Rico, it would be useful to have some clinical knowledge and skills rather than a pure laboratory background.

In the context of my research elective with you and that one publication we did together in the *Journal of Experimental Medicine*, I believe that I have moderate to high chances of getting into the residency of my choice. Because of your immense contribution in teaching and research, I would be in a much better state if you could kindly recommend me for residency training by writing a recommendation letter. I know you are busy, but it would really make a great difference in my career. I thank you for reading this e-mail and look forward to hearing from you.

Chapter 6

Your Letters of

Recommendation

The main purpose of this chapter is to familiarize you with the style or format of your LORs. This chapter can also be helpful for your LOR writers, as it shows how strongly and accurately your LORs should be presented to program directors. It is not really about how big of a person your LOR writer is (maybe partly it is for some PDs!). It is about the content, source, credibility, and your performance. The LOR writers are expected to introduce themselves within the content of the letter and should explain in what context or perspective they are commenting on your clinical skills and personal attributes.

Your LOR should speak volumes about you (succinctly though) and should not sound generic. Your LOR writers are expected to address you by your first or last name rather than simply by "he" or "she." Poorly written LORs are the ones that are generic, nonpersonalized, very short and uncertain, and with poor grammar. The letter should be signed at the bottom and preferably should be in the letter pad of the institution your LOR writer is working for. Do not forget to provide an exact address to where the letter should be sent. Some candidates provide an addressed and stamped envelope so that your letter gets on the move as soon as it has been written.

Sample Letter 1

(From a research supervisor and a physician who offered the applicant clinical observership)

Dear Program Director,

I am writing this letter of recommendation for Dr. Tanya Castro. I have been working with Dr. Castro as a research collaborator since 2007. I also supervised her while she was doing a clinical externship for the duration of three months.

I was very impressed with Dr. Castro's innovative ideas, motivation, and desire and determination to complete the work at hand. As a result of her hard work and perseverance, she has authored two abstracts, presented her work in an international meeting, and received several awards.

Apart from demonstrating a high degree of productivity and establishing a successful track record in research, Dr. Castro has continued to show her desire and determination to pursue a clinical career. This is evidenced by the fact that she passed USMLE Step 1 and Step 2 CK and CS all at the first attempt while working full-time in the research lab. After getting her ECFMG certification, Dr. Castro showed her keenness to gain some U.S. clinical experience so that she could be well prepared for the residency training. Impressed with her commitment, I created an opportunity for her to have some clinical experience at the Richardson Clinics for three months. During this period, she scrupulously took history, examined the patients, suggested differential diagnoses and the investigation plans, counseled patients, and prepared patient notes. I noticed that Dr. Castro was kind, compassionate, helpful, and respectful to the patients. She was a careful listener and demonstrated patience and professionalism. In fact, many of the patients told me that they were very pleased to have her as one of their caretakers.

She was liked not only by the patients but also by the staff members and her coworkers because of her good interpersonal and communication skills and her ability to work as a team member. She has the capability to find the point of common interest and intermingle with others very well. It took me no time to conceive why she scored very high in her medical school and received several awards. In fact, I rank her among the top 10 percent of the students that I have supervised.

I enthusiastically recommend Dr. Castro for your residency program.

Sample Letter 2

(For an applicant of pediatrics residency who has performed extremely well during medical school)

Dear Program Director,

I am writing this letter to extend my full and enthusiastic support of Dr. Vinaya Gupta's residency application in pediatrics. I am a professor of pediatrics at Case Western Reserve University School of Medicine. Dr. Gupta did a monthlong clinical clerkship under my supervision from November 2008 to December 2008, and it is within this context that I am commenting on his clinical abilities and moral attributes.

Unlike other undergraduate students, Dr. Gupta needs very little supervision. He has a habit of spending plenty of time at his patients' bedside, talking to them. One thing very striking about Dr. Gupta was his outstanding communication skills and strong sense of humor. The unique thing about Dr. Gupta is that he not only excels in patient care, but he also shows an equal passion for research. He established a sound collaboration with the neonatology division and investigated the role of CRP elevation in acute pulmonary edema. I attended a meeting where Dr. Gupta presented his work. His presentations show clarity, and he performs his work promptly. During his clerkship, Dr. Gupta clearly and consistently surpassed my expectations and stood right at the top 2 percent among his peers. He has excelled in the areas of patient care, procedural skills, availability, and communication abilities. The faculty members, including the vice chair of the pediatrics department, have graded Dr. Gupta as a superior medical student.

Dr. Gupta was also very well liked by the staff members and his coworkers because of his excellent interpersonal and communication skills and his ability to work as a team member. Perhaps more importantly, Dr. Gupta's high moral character makes him a prime candidate for the pediatrics residency program. He is a kind, compassionate, and humble person who continuously impresses me with his willingness to help others in need.

To sum up, Dr. Gupta has a rare blend of comprehensive medical knowledge, tenacity, excellent research ability, communication, and interpersonal skills. Because of Dr. Gupta's outstanding achievements and professional attributes, I have full confidence that he will be a standout in your residency program. Once again, without any reservations, I extend my strongest possible support for his application. Please contact me if I can offer any further help.

Sample Letter 3

(For an applicant for a family medicine residency who performed rather well during medical school)

Dear Program Director,

I am writing this letter to fully support Dr. Dunker's residency application in family medicine. I have served as the direct supervisor for Dr. Dunker when she completed her clerkship as well as internship in the Department of Emergency Medicine and General Practice at Vrie Universitet, Amsterdam (VUA).

I am an associate professor of emergency medicine and general practice at VUA. According to WHO, VUA ranks as one of the best medical schools in the entire Europe as it is well known for its high standards of problem-oriented medical education. As a coordinator and supervisor of several academic programs, I have had the opportunity to evaluate over 500 graduate students, including Dr. Dunker.

Dr. Dunker is a very bright physician-student with excellent interpersonal and clinical skills. Students and interns rotating in our department are required to take history, perform physical examination, order and interpret necessary laboratory tests, and institute appropriate therapeutic measures, including minor surgical procedures. Dr. Dunker excelled in all of these areas.

Because of lower doctor-to-patient ratio, tertiary-care centers like our hospital have had to bear a major flux of diverse patients. Dr. Dunker handled her patients in a kind, compassionate, and professional manner. She was humble, meticulous in her work, confident, and practical in decision making. Dr. Dunker was a very enthusiastic and motivated intern, which was evidenced by the fact that she spent extra hours working with the patients and also volunteered to help others in the Emergency Room, even during the weekends. As a result, Dr. Dunker has also learned to perform some extraclinical procedures like insertion of the chest tube and CVP line, thoracentecis, pericardiocentesis, and lumbar puncture, which are not the mandatory procedures required to be learned by the students rotating in ER.

Dr. Dunker's interpersonal skills are excellent. The other interns and staff members working with her commented favorably about her. One incident illustrates this point. There was a staff member in our department, a rather prickly person who has had some problems with medical students in the past. Dr. Dunker had to interact with this person in order to get her work properly done. She was able to find a common interest with this staff, which was horseback riding, and built a rapport based on this mutual interest. At the end of her rotation, the staff member noted what a pleasure it was to work with Dr. Dunker.

Dr. Dunker is a very determined and dedicated physician. She always liked getting engaged in clinical discussions and showed keenness in helping others in need. Because of her in-depth knowledge, motivation to teach and learn, and her good grasp of English, she was very much liked by her colleagues and many other international medical students who performed clerkship in our department.

I have no hesitation to say that Dr. Dunker is a very talented physician, whose hardworking nature, motivation, and determination have pushed her to the very top among her peers. I have no doubt that she will excel in every health care team she joins in the future. I wish her good luck in her future career.

Sample Letter 4

(For an applicant who has been out of medical school for a while)

Dear Program Director,

I am writing this letter to strongly support Dr. Emily Adeoba's residency application. Dr. Adeoba recently informed me of her interest in joining a residency program in your department and asked if I could provide her a reference. Though it has already been a while since we worked together, it does not take me a minute to recall her abilities as the impressions she had made on me are as carved in stone.

I am a professor working in the Emergency Department of Southern Tripolo University. Being a staff member of a teaching hospital, I am allocated to supervise medical students and interns. I had had an opportunity to evaluate the abilities and future potential of Dr. Adeoba when she rotated to our department as a senior medical student as well as an intern for the period of one and a half months.

Dr. Adeoba is a strong team player and a committed professional who has an in-depth medical knowledge, excellent clinical and interpersonal skills, a good grasp of English, and a very calm, compassionate, and soothing personality.

Dr. Adeoba is an innovative self-starter, who rarely needs supervision. Dr. Adeoba was one of the best interns, who fulfilled her responsibilities in a very professional and efficient manner. She was meticulous in taking history, examining patients, composing a differential diagnosis, ordering suitable lab tests, and formulating a treatment plan. I have received many compliments from the patients who relied on her care. Nurses, staff, and other students praise her working abilities.

Dr. Adeoba bears superior skills and excellent work ethics. She is punctual and typically exceeds expectations. She strictly adheres to hospital standards and guidelines, handles pressure well, and voluntarily works overtime. I just recall one instance when Dr. Adeoba worked as an intern in the Emergency Room (ER). There are usually one staff (attending), one resident, and two interns who cover the ER of our hospital on a night shift. One day, the staff and one of the interns both could not make it to the hospital for some personal reasons, leaving the resident and Dr. Adeoba alone to cover the busy night shift. Dr. Adeoba worked in such an efficient and professional manner that the resident who worked with her told me the next morning that she was one of the best interns he had ever worked with. He was very pleased with Dr. Adeoba's performance. Even the head of the department and other staff members were very impressed with her abilities. This is just one example among many of Dr. Adeoba's superior skills and admirable work ethics.

Dr. Adeoba is an invaluable asset to any health care team, and I highly recommend recruiting her. If you'd like to discuss her attributes in more detail, please don't hesitate to contact me.

Sample Letter 5

(From a professor who worked with an applicant only briefly but still wants to help)

Dear Program Director,

I am a professor of nephrology and a former director of the Institute of Urology and Nephrology in Southern University of Michigan. This hospital is a highly advanced tertiary-care facility dedicated to advanced clinical care, teaching, and research.

Dr. Miller did a clinical externship directly under my supervision from January 2008 to April 2008. Right from the beginning, I was highly impressed with his level of motivation, sound medical knowledge, and his ability to garner these components for making appropriate clinical decisions. I provided him the opportunity to take history, perform physical exam, and formulate a management plan in patients with several medical problems. Dr. Miller also rotated through our dialysis and kidney transplantation facility. In a short time, Dr. Miller convinced me that he has excellent medical knowledge, skills, and aptitude to learn and improve.

To summarize, Dr. Miller is a very dedicated clinician with substantial clinical experience, and is expected to perform very well in the clinics. I strongly support his desires and determination to join a physician scientist training pathway in your facility. I predict that Dr. Miller will be one of your dependable and industrious residents, and I wish him well in the future.

If you need any information, please do not hesitate to e-mail me.

Chapter 7

The Status of Your

Application

Once you apply for your residency through ERAS, it is not common to e-mail programs about how your application is doing. The main reason behind this is that programs receive thousands of applications for a limited number of training positions they offer. You may choose to write them if there is a significant change in the status of your application. For example, if you have started a clinical clerkship in a local hospital, then it may help to let the program know. If you have been working on a research paper that just got accepted to a cool peer-reviewed journal, then this is the time to write the program. Some candidates may also want to update the program about their USMLE results (like Step 3). Utilizing this opportunity to write them, you can also ask the PD about the status of your application. Remember, most of the time, these issues are handled by program coordinators, and do not be surprised if you receive a generic e-mail stating, "We are still reviewing your application and will get back to you in the near future."

Sample 1

(This program was hesitant to give an interview—at least until this e-mail was sent.)

Dear Dr. Vincent:

I have recently applied to your program for a residency position through ERAS. You will notice from my personal statement that I am highly interested and motivated to pursue a career in pathology. I understand that pathology is a highly competitive specialty and that it requires a lot of homework to secure a spot for training.

In the past years, I have carefully prepared myself to become eligible for getting residency training in this field. After graduating from medical school, I have gained two years of research experience in cardiorenal pathology and molecular biology. In this period, I have not only learned useful laboratory skills such as immunohistochemistry, flow cytometry, gene amplification and real-time PCR, cell culture, etc., but I have also developed excellent presentation and communication skills by participating in various research meetings and national and international conferences. On top of that, I have also familiarized myself with U.S. clinical setup by doing clinical rotation in Belle Clinic.

As a result of perseverance, self-reliance, dedication, and the ability to work as a team member, I have excelled very well in my area of research and have published three research articles in peer-reviewed and highly cited international journals. However, my dream of making a direct contribution in patient care while keeping abreast of academic medicine can only come true if I get training in pathology in a world-class institution like yours. Therefore, I am requesting you to consider my candidacy for your program.

Thank you so much for your attention, and I look forward to hearing from you soon.

Example 2

(There was some delay in the interview invitation from this program, but not after this e-mail was sent.)

Dear Dr. Smart:

Hope you are well and having an interesting resident recruitment season. I understand that you receive an overwhelming number of applications for PGY-1 openings and you might still have to review mine.

After interviewing with you last year, I have continuously dedicated my time and efforts to addressing your concerns regarding my candidacy. Right after I returned to New York from Michigan, I started my clinical externship at Newington Clinic under the supervision of the clinic director. During externship, I had ample opportunity to interact with patients with diverse medical problems. I also used this opportunity to familiarize myself with state-of-the art computer programs like care plus and CPRS. I was very much liked by my patients, who complimented my care as being "full of compassion and love."

I know dreaming of getting into your residency program is not easy to make a reality, but I am confident that I will take excellent care of my patients and have more to offer for cutting-edge clinical research. I am extremely impressed with the openness, diversity, flexibility, and academic rigor of your training program and would like to choose Michigan as my place for further training.

While I write this e-mail, please allow me to update you that I have just passed USMLE Step 3 (94th percentile). Currently, I am revising MKSAP in order to consolidate my clinical knowledge.

I sincerely hope that my credentials meet your expectations. I am eagerly anticipating your decision regarding my application.

Chapter 8

Residency Interview

It is very important to have a clear understanding of the residency interview process before you actually attend one. Remember, the early bird catches the worm. So schedule your interviews early enough. Once you know your interview date, work on your flight and hotel accommodations. It is convenient to stay close to the hospital you are going to interview at. The evening before the interview, many programs will invite you for dinner. Most of the time, these dinners are attended by senior residents or chief residents. However, some programs have their faculty members come in to such pre-interview dinners. The pre-interview dinner is a unique opportunity to sense the atmosphere and determine whether this particular program would be the best fit for you.

Realize that pre-interview dinner is not an actual interview. Make yourself comfortable, order a familiar menu, drink in moderation (if you choose to), and ask reasonable and natural questions (for example, you do not need to know the nationalities of individual residents). Instead, questions like how frequent are the in-house calls, who gives the conferences, are there dedicated research electives, etc., constitute common but natural questions. You can also ask about the neighborhood, housing, schools, etc., based on your personal interests and circumstances. Some candidates like to discuss baseball, soccer, basketball, etc., but make sure your counterpart is familiar with the topics you are getting into. Overall, be simplistic rather than complex, be human than superhuman, be down-to-earth rather than up the air. You are applying for internship; and a successful intern would be friendly, eager to learn, and will be committed to the scholarship. More than anything else, a great intern would be a dependable physician and a dedicated learner and educator.

Common Interview Questions

It is hard to predict what questions the interviewer will have in mind. In general, interview questions are divided into the following components:

1. Introduction
2. Education, research, and any other academic qualifications
3. Candidate's goals, objectives, and future plans
4. Any personal interests or hobbies
5. Personality, communication skills, clinical knowledge
6. Any questions candidates can have about the program

During your interview, your interviewer is not supposed to go into the questions listed below. However, if they step out of the norms, you still are expected to answer them in a professional manner. Do not appear frustrated; it is you who needs to get into the residency training.

The interviewers should not be asking you the following questions:

1. What is your nationality?
2. What is your religious belief?
3. How old are you?
4. How many children do you have?
5. Are you disabled?

Below are the common interview questions you will encounter. Remember, there is no best or worst answer for any question. Try avoiding statements like "I disagree," "I would agree with you if . . ." Absorb some criticisms while defend yourself for others. Just like a normal human being, like yourself or any of your colleagues.

Tell me about yourself.

This question is, surprisingly, quite common. Although this is widely open ended and does not specifically fit into the objective of residency interview, many interviewers like asking this question because it's easy to ask and can be a reasonable icebreaker. There is no hard-and-fast rule to answering this question, and certainly, this question is *not* about telling the interviewer your name, date of birth, visa status, USMLE scores, etc. Use the following strategy to answer this question:

1. One introductory sentence about who you are

2. One sentence about your qualifications

3. One sentence about your experience

4. One or two sentences about what you would like to do in the future

Sample answer: I am a medical school graduate from Iceland with a master's degree from the University of London, England. During this course, I have faced several transitions in life: transition in geography, in the way patient care is done, in education and professional advancement. I love what I am doing and am determined to learn and improve. I intend to pursue a career in internal medicine and continue doing research in the area of diabetes-induced kidney diseases. In the future, I see myself as a competent physician with high professional and moral standards.

Why did you choose this specialty?

It is natural and common for the programs to ask you why you want to pursue a career in that particular field. I know we all have our thoughts and reasons. Certainly it depends on what we prioritize in life. For many of us, it is based on what our underlying circumstances dictate us to embrace as a career choice. Your answers to such questions should be logical and insightful. Learning opportunities, diversity of patient population, flexible lifestyle, above-average professional satisfaction, research opportunities, etc., constitute the common reasons why you would like to pursue one field over the other. However, financial reimbursement, family or peer pressure, and looking to do anything I can, etc., although true in many occasions, are not highly appreciated answers, at least during the course of your interview.

Examples

Why do you want to do internal medicine residency?

There are different areas of internal medicine, and each of them is very interesting.

Internists care: We care for patients with chest pain, trouble breathing, leg swelling, dementia, and so forth. We have a broad concept of comprehensive and rather holistic approach to patient care. This makes internal medicine a unique and well-sought-after specialty.

Internal medicine is rewarding: Internists impact their patient's life in a positive way and establish long-term relationships. For example, it is highly rewarding when you convince your patient to quit smoking. It is gratifying when you diagnose an ignored case of diabetic neuropathy. It just gets more and more interesting every day. It inspires me when I am able to help my patients and their family members.

Above-average professional satisfaction: Last but not the least, I have spoken to several practicing internists regarding their professional satisfaction and how they have balanced their personal and family life. They unanimously expressed above-average personal and professional satisfaction, which has further enhanced my desire to develop a sound career in internal medicine.

Why do you want to do pathology residency?

A successful treatment begins with a correct diagnosis. Needless to say, pathology is a medical specialty that provides the basic foundation for all medical practices. Pathology has been the field of medicine I liked the most since my early days in medical school. *Robbins Pathologic Basis of Disease* used to be my favorite textbook, and I used to read it every single day. Besides playing a critical role in disease diagnosis and patient care, a pathologist can serve as an educator and researcher, and that perfectly fits into my career objectives. Pathologists have a unique advantage in biomedical research because of their close ties to clinical medicine, their familiarity with laboratory techniques, and their insight into the significance of diseased tissue changes.

What is your weakness?

Sure, we all have weaknesses in life. Some of us have had a heavy Saturday night that got us into trouble the next morning. Many of us have had an argument with our girl/boyfriends at some point of our life. It is natural, and it reflects we are human beings. Your residency interview is not about revealing all these weaknesses; neither can you fool the PDs by stating, "My biggest weakness is that I work too hard." Some candidates add an element of humor to this question and gently deflect it. Others want to answer it in a rather diplomatic way.

Sample answer: My three-year-old niece thinks my weakness is that I cannot remember all her nursery rhymes and that is true. Anyway, to answer your question, when I engage myself in a very emotional conversation pertaining to life and death with my patients or their family, I tend to forget that they are not my family members. I tend to be very emotional. However, with time and experience, this is getting better.

What are your strengths?

Again, residency interview is not the occasion you would like to rave about your strengths. They already have your credentials, including USMLE scores and the dean's letter. You have already stated in your application whether you have received any awards or honors. Your publications are listed in your common application form. So the bottom line is they know you. The answer to this question, at the minimum, should not go wrong. Your answer should be correct and actually match your strength. If you say critical thinking and scientific interrogation are your strengths, the next question will be, "What have you achieved so far out of this unique asset you own?"

Sample answer: There is nothing like a stone-set strength in my life, and there is no known gray area where I fear to buckle up because that is not my strongest area. I think what I am now is a reflection of what I have learned in different stages of my life and how I have shaped my future. However, I would consider punctuality and humbleness as two of my biggest strengths. I would lose everything else before I lose these two proud assets of my life.

Why are you interested in this program?

This is an extremely common question and requires some homework on your part to answer it appropriately. Here comes the relevance of doing some research about the program, faculties, residents, and chief residents before you actually attend the interview. Find out what is unique about the program you are interviewing for, sense the atmosphere of academics vs. private practice, dig into the research interests of the faculty members, and at least go over the abstracts of the manuscripts written by the people who are going to interview you. If you already know someone working there, remember to call that person at least the night before. Get familiar with local weather, people's interests, and even sports teams, if you can.

Generic answer: I hope to become part of a residency program that is endowed with an academically productive and supportive environment. I wish to become a part of a medical team that is dedicated to patient care as well as teaching and research. Your program will provide me this opportunity.

Focused answer: This program has some important characteristics that other programs lack. This hospital, located in a busy inner-city neighborhood, has a big volume and diversity of patients. On the other hand, your Individual Resident Mentorship approach is unique in the sense that I will have a goal-directed training and one-to-one mentorship. Furthermore, I have compelling family reasons to stay around this area as far as possible. I have revised the highlights of your program, and your program best fits my interest.

How does your past experience enhance your ability to become a successful resident?

This is a rather straightforward question. You have to explain what you did in the past and how the knowledge and experience you acquired will help you to become a successful resident. For example, if you spent six months in Madrid learning Spanish, you acquired an additional skill of communicating directly with a Spanish-speaking population.

Sample answer: During my past training, I have gained significant experience in patient care, teaching, and clinical research. As a rotating intern working in tertiary-care center, I had had access to examine and care for a large volume of patients with diverse diseases, which allowed me to develop sound clinical skills. My past experience has helped me develop qualities that are essential for the practice of medicine. My hard work and motivation to learn have enabled me to develop a broad foundation of knowledge and scientific background. My service on the Medical Student Organization as a representative and my training as an MS student helped me to foster my leadership, decision-making, and communication skills. My experience of traveling to diverse regions has allowed me to learn about new cultures and experience the world. This will allow me to understand and take care of patients from diverse communities.

What are your goals and objectives?

This is probably the most important question you will be asked during your interview. If you do not know what your weaknesses are, you will still be up and hitting. If you do not know your goals (both short-term as well as long-term), you are at a huge disadvantage. Not having a goal equals to not having a vision, or even the desire, to do a residency. Always spell out your goals in your personal statement and get ready to reiterate and defend them during your interview.

Sample answer: I want to be able to build my life to include both a fulfilling career in pediatrics as well as time dedicated to being a husband and a father. Obviously, my first goal is to develop clinical skills that will enable me to work as an independent thinker and decision maker. However, I am also passionate about teaching and research.

Ten years from today, I see myself as a successful pediatrician who has gained the confidence of his patients and his colleagues. Although the entire field of pediatrics is very interesting for me at this stage, the area of pediatric cardiology intrigues me the most.

In conclusion, the interview questions have no borders or limitations. If you are interviewing in an academic center, majority of the interview questions will be teaching and research oriented. If you are interviewing in a community hospital, your questions will be more inclined toward primary care, patient diversity, patient volume, etc. It is not uncommon for them to ask you to describe a clinical case scenario that you encountered. Always have a simple, common, but intriguing case presentation in your mind. Finally, just relax and enjoy your interview trail; interviews are not meant to be scary ordeals. They are actually designed to meet the goals common to you and your potential training program.

Chapter 9

Thank-You Letters

Thank-you letters do not constitute the main or vital component of residency selection. For a large program that interviews hundreds of candidates, it can be almost impossible to go over individual thank-you letters. However, do not get surprised if they respond to your letter with a very personal and live e-mail stating how much the faculty enjoyed meeting with you. So, the bottom line is to send a thank-you note. Thank-you letters are to be sent sooner rather than later (preferably within a day, and not later than a week).

Your thank-you letter should be personal, specific to what you discussed during the interview, and should embrace what you particularly liked about the program, city, or people. Do not write statements like "I am planning to rank your program right at the top." Instead, write "Because of its clinical and academic excellence, diversity of training experience, and plenty of research opportunities, I am sure your program gets the first preference over others."

In summary, thank-you letters are meant to thank the faculty, residents, fellows, and other supporting staff who have provided you this opportunity for a residency interview. Thank them, be grateful to them, and show your enthusiasm. Do not be discouraged if you do not receive a response. Do not write multiple thank-you notes to one person. Be patient and remain optimistic.

Thank-you letter 1

Dear Dr. Normandy,

I would like to sincerely thank you for taking the time to educate me about your program and also for letting me express my desire and determination to join your residency training. I particularly enjoyed the pre-interview dinner and sharing some stories about Spain with you. I spoke to Ricky on the interview day and learned more about your current projects. The entire process was extraordinarily well organized, and faculties were enthusiastic to help me achieve my future goals and objectives. At the end of the day, when the interviews were over, all my questions were answered.

Dr. Normandy, I know your program is highly competitive and attracts many accomplished physicians from all over the nation. Indeed, I have tremendous respect and regard for your program. However, I have worked very hard while remaining motivated, focused, and goal oriented. As an early career physician scientist looking to enhance both research and clinical skills, I strongly believe your place would be the best fit for me. If you have any additional queries about my application, I would be more than happy to travel back to your place and have a second conversation with you. Once again, thank you so much for your support, and I look forward to working with you.

Thank-you letter 2

Dear Dr. Tang,

I would like to sincerely thank you for taking the time to educate me about your clinical work and research, and also for letting me express my desire and determination to join your program. I had a very unique and gratifying experience on the day of the interview. In particular, I enjoyed sharing the news and events about my past experience of doing research in Alabama and discussing the novel molecules: PPAR and Citrullin. More interestingly, your imaging-based data on MI were fascinating.

Dr. Tang, after visiting your program and having a daylong experience of meeting accomplished and inspiring faculty members, my interest in joining your program has only intensified. I truly believe that your training program can help facilitate the fulfillment of my dreams. Once again, thank you, and I look forward to meeting you in the future.

Thank-you letter 3

Dear Dr. Moulton,

I hope you are well and having a productive resident recruitment season. It was a great pleasure interviewing with you last Thursday. I very much appreciate you and your staff allotting so much of your time to talk with me about the details of your program. I firmly believe that training offered in MIC perfectly meets my educational objectives and goals.

I particularly liked the diverse training offered in academic hospitals as well as in community-based hospitals, the diverse background of the staff, the resident and patient population, and the openness of the program. Above all, I am very much impressed with the abundance of highly qualified faculty members who are experienced diagnosticians, researchers, and gifted teachers.

Obviously, Dr. Moulton, my first and foremost priority at this stage is to get the training that arms me with diagnostic competence in pathology. However, I am equally passionate about research and teaching. I have understood that I would not have too much spare time to perform bench research during residency. Given the caveat, I would be more than happy to participate in some of the ongoing research projects under the mentorship of an experienced faculty member without compromising my training. We certainly will sit down together and discuss this exciting opportunity in the near future. I am very hopeful that I stand up to the expectations of MIC and will land a residency position.

Again, Dr. Moulton, thank you so much for your time. If you have any questions about my qualifications or personal attributes, please feel free to contact me.

Chapter 10

Addressing PD's

Concerns

It is not unusual for program directors, even with the best intentions, to have some concerns about your current application or previous training. Most of the time, these issues are addressed during the interview. If a PD writes you an e-mail with specific concerns, that is considered to be a good sign, as long as your response is adequate and appropriate to address the PD's concerns. Be mindful of the length of your e-mail. An extremely long e-mail gathers no extra points but risks getting deleted without someone reading it. Be succinct, direct; and address the PD's actual concern. Do not divert the issue, and do not keep on reminding the PD about your USMLE scores. They know how well you have done.

Depending on the nature of their question, you can get some help from your mentor or your dean. It is not a great idea to call the PD if he or she has not shown such intent in the e-mail you have received. Program coordinators can be a lot of help if you have not understood the question very well. If the question is related to your visa status, either get some help from someone who knows more about it, or carefully check the following website: www.uscis.gov.

Example

(In this case, the program director was not sure whether this candidate could work well in the U.S. health care setting.)

Dear Dr. Brown:

Thank you so much for your e-mail. I truly appreciate your interest in my application. One thing I like the most about this interview trail is that I get to know so many individuals from different walks of life. Over the month of October, I traveled to many places in the USA, met several candidates with diverse trainings and interests. Dr. Brown, as you stated in your e-mail, there are certain aspects of the U.S. health care system that I need to learn and get used to, at least during the first couple of months of my internship. However, when it comes to determination to work hard, learn, improve, and advance the science, I have found myself quite at par with many other residency candidates I have met recently. My clinical training in my home country and my track record of doing research in U.S. health care settings and U.S. clinical experience conducted during my three-month-long clinical observership in your hospital are some of the assets that will be helpful when I work in an inner-city hospital like yours. In addition, I will devote a substantial amount of time and effort to enhance my research skills. I strongly feel the University of South Montana is a right fit for me.

Dr. Brown, I hope I have addressed your concerns. Thank you for your support, and I look forward to working with you in the near future.

Chapter 11

After the Match Results

Years of hard work, determination, and perseverance to pursue your dream will certainly lead to joy and happiness on Match Day. Enjoy the great news; call your parents and let your friends know how happy you are. Your next step is to apply for a medical license to practice medicine and get ready to move to the place you matched. Your residency program will send a thick package to your home address within a week or so. So if you have changed your address, give them a call to update your contact details.

If you did not match, this is certainly not the end of the era. You did not match this year, but you still have chances the following years! Retrospectively, try to figure out why you did not get enough interview calls. If you interviewed with several programs but still did not match, try to understand why you were not ranked high enough. Did you remember to certify your rank order list? For international medical graduates, common concerns are U.S. clinical experience, number of years away from medical school, communication and linguistic skills, etc. Local graduates do also face similar challenges, but U.S. clinical experience is not a matter of concern for them.

Remember, there are a fair number of residency positions available through the post-match scramble process. Even after the scramble, be alert as to whether the program has an unexpected opening of a residency slot. If you feel comfortable writing some PDs about your situation, it may not be a bad idea since they have more time to read your e-mail. If nothing else works, start preparing your application for the next residency recruitment season. Good luck.

This e-mail saved someone a year!

Dear Dr. Beermann,

I am writing this e-mail to inquire about a residency position at your facility. I recently visited your university hospital and had an opportunity to familiarize myself with the essence of your program structure. It took me no time to decide that your program would be an ideal place where I could fulfill my ever-growing need for developing a sound career as an internist.

After two years of basic science and clinical research, I have wished to start my clinical career with a decisive outlook and a resolute mind. During my research, I have found striking similarities between basic science research and clinical practice: both would need determination, perseverance, and an evidence-based approach. Internal medicine spans a very broad field of clinical care. Because of its expansive reach for patient care, education, and research, it has become the subject of first preference for me. I have learned that your program has an outstanding track for patient care, medical education, and clinical research, making it an attractive target to choose.

Getting enrolled into your program is my primary goal, also due to the fact that my fiancé, Mike Peterson, is already doing his residency with you. Regarding my academic eligibility, I have passed USMLE Step 1 and Step 2 CK and CS all in my first attempt and I have gained some U.S. clinical experience to familiarize myself with the U.S. health care system. I am eligible for temporary licensure and do not require a visa (I am a permanent U.S. resident). Since I already hold a valid ECFMG certificate, finding a residency for this academic session could save me a year.

Therefore, I am requesting you to consider my candidacy if a residency training position becomes available in your program. I believe that you will find me as one of the most motivated and dedicated residents.

Thank you so much for your consideration, and I look forward to hearing from you.

Dallas → PA.
Cancell 120$
change

PA → Dallas.

→ coolmaies.co
→ zzstream.u

Rochester General has
less than 5 miles
do a

Nelo
9820143677

one night
3rd December
ID 2 clean non smo
Breakfast
free wifi
check in : 8 3:00
checkout : after noon
Elizabeth
6556668

→ Black **Zara** dress
→ Big leather dress
→ alter purple lacy dress
→ Mango blazer
→ see other formal dresses
→ sewing material
→ waxing material

Raja Tatha

PS73

Made in the USA
Lexington, KY
01 November 2011